CONSCIOUS I

An Invitation to Intuitive Nourishment

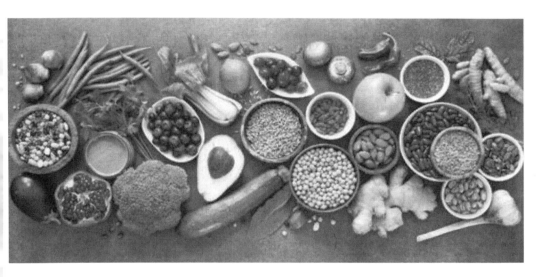

by

Shaun de Warren & Brian Mayne

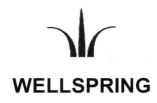

WELLSPRING

Acknowledgements

We would like to acknowledge our original Conscious Eating Group that initiated this project several years ago, and particularly Katya Forner who was instrumental in inspiring the idea of turning this group's findings into a book. We also acknowledge the more recent Conscious Eating Groups and individuals who met at The Centre in Battersea to explore these principles further and to report on their findings. Thanks go to Gill de Warren and Geeta Patel who checked the text and advised on layout and design. Finally, we would like to acknowledge the originator of the four principles, whomever that was, on which our explorations here are based.

Please note (medical caution and disclaimer)

The authors do not dispense medical advice or prescribe the use of the principles and information in this book as forms of treatment for sickness without medical approval. Nutritionists and other experts in the field of health and nutrition hold widely varying views. In the event you use information from this publication without your doctor's approval, you are prescribing for yourself. That is your right, but the publisher and authors assume no responsibility.

CONTENTS

INTRODUCTION

A group of us, dissatisfied with diets and confused by what all the "experts" say on what we should and should not eat, came together to explore a different way ...a way directed from within and a way which trusts that the body knows what it wants and needs if we truly listen to it.

Our group expanded into more than one and these were made up of different individuals with a variety of occupations: management consultant, publisher, author, counsellor, university professor, graphic designer, performer, beauty therapist, financial controller, mothers and homemakers (of both sexes) among others.

The challenge our group immediately perceived was that our mind and emotions call for all sorts of foods, some of which we know are not of the highest true value (and some of which not only have no value whatsoever, but which may actually be destructive to our health and well-being). We were aware that these were the calls of the mind and emotions, rather than of the body. Similarly, although not as usual, instead of calling for food, some people's minds and emotions deny food to their bodies. Both of these extremes can result in damage to physical health, all kinds of illness and even death.

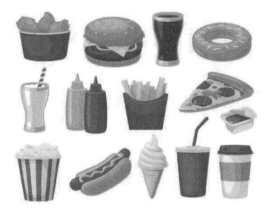

Conscious eating is about becoming aware of the call of the body, which speaks to us intuitively, rather than through the mind or emotions. The body, we discovered, calls for love and for nutrition created from love. The mind and emotions are subject to habit, compulsion and addiction, which are not love.

A distinction arose, therefore, between satisfying the true call of the body and recognising what were merely mental and emotional cravings, compensations and addictions. Although addictions can give us valuable information about ourselves, they want further exploration to discover the real issues underlying them and what may be true nourishment for us.

Thus we embarked on our journey, basing it on four simple principles we had discovered. They are not original, and we acknowledge whomever it was who brought them to light. These principles are anchored in the One Principle: love is all there is, and this we see to be the first and greatest principle in life.

We invite you to participate in this experiment and we recommend you try the programme included here. Each stage of it is intended to inspire, support and take you to deeper and deeper levels of exploring what conscious eating means for you. Please treat them in a fun way and not as a rigorous discipline. Include them in your daily living in a way that is enjoyable and which works for you.

We also suggest that if you do the programme, you do it with a friend or with a group of friends. It can be fun to share your individual experiences, as we did, and having a support group can really make a difference to your commitment and results. At the end of each chapter, we include comments and findings about it, which came from our groups.

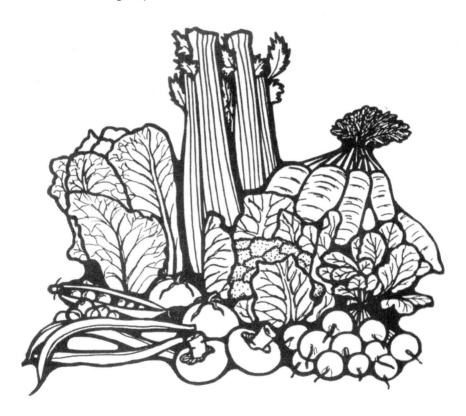

CHAPTER 1

The Four Principles

Our self-exploration is based on the four principles of conscious eating:

1. Eat when we are hungry.

2. Eat what we love.

3. Love what we eat.

4. Stop when we have had enough.

What lies behind the principles of conscious eating is that if we really eat what we love and love what we eat, we will be in very good health, because we will naturally want to eat things which are nourishing for the body and which contribute to our energy level and sense of well-being.

The four principles ask us to listen to our bodies, rather than to the interpretations of our minds and emotions. The 'we,' or 'you,' they refer to is in that feeling/awareness/beingness place inside which precedes anything you think about.

Our group's findings are by no means final on this subject, but a beginning of a process of personal exploration and continuous refinement for us. This book is for you to benefit from these findings so far and to allow you to commence your own individual exploration.

What if all our eating is based on the principle of love? This would mean an end to the struggling, an end to the dieting and an end to the self-torture we heap upon ourselves when we "fail," along with the resulting loss in self-esteem.

What if love is the way?

Each of you embarking on this venture becomes your own laboratory. Exploring these principles is exploring yourself and establishing a new relationship with eating. Each of you is your own tester in eating, your own scientist, and your own expert.

Food is nature's physical way of providing cosmic energy to fuel the body. The key is the energy, rather than the food - which is a medium. Conscious eating is not so much about the quantities or specific kinds of food you eat, but rather about the extent to which what you eat refuels, re-energises, and revitalises your body.

"Aha!" say the 'experts', "You need vitamins, proteins, fibre, etc."

"Maybe," we say, "but when we listen to the body, it tells us what it wants".

We find out for ourselves what the body is calling for and how best to satisfy it. We have done away with experts and their 'answers,' and we have done away with diets, both of which control us from the outside and both of which we often associate with denial. We have given ourselves permission to trust our senses (notably our intuition) and to find out for ourselves what looks great, what smells great, what tastes great and what makes us feel great.

Diets are things we come off as soon as possible (if not sooner)! Conscious eating is self-discipline and is for life. It is about being natural and non-judgemental about foods.

Conscious eating says:
"I love myself!"
"I love my body!"
"I love the food I eat!"
"Nutrition (which means receiving ...in all its forms) is one of the highest ways we can align with Divine energy."

Our Experiences and Comments

Shaun:
- The Conscious eating programme works for me as a framework within which to explore my relationship with food and eating. It gives me a list of useful questions to ask myself:

Gill:
- I set out on the Conscious Eating programme with the intention of becoming aware of what I eat, and of being more conscious of foods that will be good for me to eat at any given time. I would also like to improve my level of energy in order to keep up a sometimes-fast lifestyle.

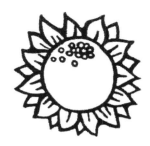

CHAPTER 2

Eat When We Are Hungry

Each of us has a hunger barometer that can give us a 'zero' to 'ten' reading on our hunger level. If the barometer is at 'five,' we are feeling fine, not hungry, and not in need of any food. We are just feeling good. If the barometer's at 'four,' we could eat a little bit. If it is at 'one', we are starving, which is unlikely for almost everyone in the Western world. If we are at 'nine,' it means we are so bloated we can't move, perhaps such as after a festive meal or similar blowout. Most Westerners probably only hit 'nine' once or twice a year. 'Eight' is definitely full, a feeling of "I don't think I want to eat again for the rest of the week." 'Seven' is a sense of being just a little bit more than satisfied, while 'six' is a nice, full feeling.

Many don't know what conscious hunger feels like, as they are always moving between a 5 and an 8 (or higher!). Others have a fear of being hungry (especially when this is associated with psychological and emotional pain and might previously have led them to obsessive compulsive eating as a way of lessening this pain). For these cases, it might be helpful to have a 'Hunger Day' (a day's fast), just to find out what hunger feels like.

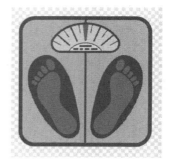

We can begin reading this hunger barometer and using it more consciously. Very extreme cases, like anorexics, may only eat (if at all) when they hit 'two,' or even 'one.' What many of us tend to do, though, is to treat 'five' as if it were 'zero,' so that, when we drop back to level 'five' we think, "I need food!" and we fill ourselves up to a level of about 'seven' or 'eight.' Many people tend always to be living between levels 'five' and 'eight,' rather than from a range of between 'three' and 'six,' or 'three' and 'seven.'

Trust and eat in the moment – even if eating for comfort -, *but do it as consciously as possible*, this allows you – in the moment – to discern whether it is true hunger (physiological) or the subtle (or not so subtle) ego. Whichever you find it to be, it is important that no judgement follow. Rather, pat yourself on the back for staying conscious and for being able to distinguish between the body's and the ego's calls. The more conscious you become, the more you will automatically move to healing old destructive patterns and tend to an increasingly natural health and lifestyle.

If we truly check our body's hunger barometers, we will find that we are often not actually hungry. It is psychological (mental/emotional/ego) habit that invariably calls for food, rather than true hunger, the real call of the body. True hunger is a pleasant sensation of wanting food, as opposed to the habits of "It's breakfast time, lunchtime, dinnertime, 'time to eat' time, 'I can't think of anything else to do now' time, or 'I always eat something when I come into the kitchen' time.

We set up the patterns that ring a little chord in the cells of the body which have a memory, like the one that - for years - you have had something with your tea at this time of day. REAL hunger is NOT habit. REAL hunger is checking the barometer to see whether we are operating from 'five' to 'ten' or from 'zero' to 'ten.'

Our Experiences and Comments

Shaun
- Often, I am not hungry and realize that my eating has an emotional base quite apart from hunger; "I'm bored," "I'm tired," "It's lunchtime," "The person I'm with wants to eat and I don't want to disappoint or to set myself apart."

-The wisdom of the body - the body knows - it's grown itself and functions miraculously often in spite of how we treat it!

Brian
- I like having the growing awareness of my body's 'hunger barometer,' but have also come to learn that there are exceptions when it can be better to override it. So, sometimes it can be better to eat from an emotion's call, to acknowledge a friend's offering of food or even to ignore the body's call and follow a higher call to fast for a while. However, as a rule, I have found the body's call the best overall guide.

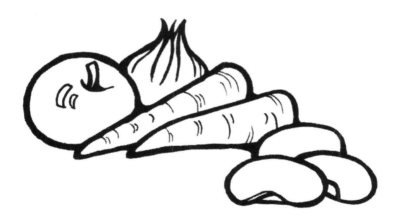

CHAPTER 3

Eat What We Love

The second principle is "Eat what we love." Normally, we eat what we think we ought to eat, or eat what we think we love, but when we are just shoving food in and swallowing it, we don't really know whether we love it or not. As we experimented, we found many of the things we had THOUGHT we loved didn't actually either taste great or make us feel good. They were not as nourishing, as exciting or as full of energy as we had thought they were.

Eating what we love eating means retraining ourselves to eat foods which are number 'tens' for us, or those that are high on the scale of 'zero' to 'ten' in terms of look, flavour/taste, quality, nourishment, how they feel in our mouth and swallowing and the vitality we receive from them. But no such list is fixed. The most important part of being clear on what your body loves is to stay connected with it and be spontaneous to its call.

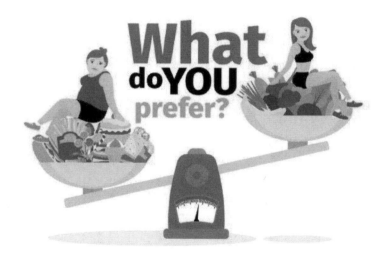

With this principle, we retrain ourselves to enjoy all of the things we love eating. Many of these foods were not on our menus because we thought they were fattening, bad for us, too expensive, or out of season. The adventure was to explore them all and find the foods we really LOVE to eat. The test question is: "Do I love it, or don't I love it?" ...and the answer comes from the body.

When we started this experiment a number of us found we were swallowing our food without checking whether we loved it. We wanted to get things down quickly, so we could get on to the pudding or whatever was next. We realised that to find out which foods we really loved, it was important to shift our attention from our minds to our bodies - "How does my body react to this food? Do I feel better after eating it, or do I feel low or worse?"

Even though we said we loved eating, when we looked more closely, we often found that what we were really saying was, "I love swallowing," "I love getting it in fast," or "I love feeling full." We weren't enjoying eating it at all, and often didn't see or know what we were eating. It just went in and, if someone were to ask us half an hour later what we had for lunch, we would have difficulty remembering. It was just a lump in our stomach. Heaven forbid someone should ask us what we had eaten for dinner yesterday, the day before or two days ago! We found that watching television, or being engaged in some other activity, while eating helped us forget what we were putting into our bodies and encouraged us to shove it in unconsciously.

Throwing things into the stomach to get a full feeling is not conscious eating. It has to do with filling an emptiness, which is something else altogether. If we are filling emptiness's, it is better for us to examine why we feel empty. What in our lives seems empty? What other forms of nourishment are we starved of (see more on this in the chapter on The Essence of Nutrition) and how can we fill the emptiness of THOSE, rather than filling up and going unconscious to them.

Initially, it helped us to write down a guide list of the foods we really love, so that we could have a reminder of what we really enjoyed and make our selections from it. As we kept adding to our list, we found there are hundreds of wonderful flavours and foods that are nourishing to us. Conscious eating is in no way a sacrifice, but an invitation to a feast we had previously not been aware of. We began to appreciate that there are thousands of foods, although in the West many of us may often enjoy less than a hundred.

Often, we realised that what we had thought was a call for food was really a call for emotional nourishment - love, intimacy, connection, touch or acknowledgement - and that filling this call with food was only a temporary solution that did not really answer the call correctly. We found that we often used some foods (such as chocolates, starchy or spicy foods) as 'fixes,' rather than as foods. Cravings, when psychological, generally indicate a 'fix,' rather than a food. This raises the larger issue of emotional and spiritual nourishment, upon which we touch later.

Learning to eat consciously became more than a food programme. It became a pleasing explanation and expansion of our own state of consciousness. We found that the body is a vibratory energy, that food is a vibratory energy and that finding the harmony in both of these can be a wonderful adventure.

Part of our conscious evolutionary process is getting back into a relationship with ourselves, with our body's vibratory energy and with the vibratory energy we put into it.

The real conscious enjoyment of food happens in the mouth and in one's feeling of well being afterward. Once food is in the stomach it follows an automatic and instinctive digestive process, which is beyond most individuals' conscious awareness.

Our Experiences and Comments

Harriet and Brian
- We see food allergies and intolerances as messengers. What are the payoffs for having them? What do I not have to do? To whom am I sending a message?

Brian
- I used to think champagne had a great value but discovered in the 'here and now' experience that I actually didn't like it very much (but had based my previous estimation of it on other people's ideas, feelings or experiences of it, rather than on my own). The experience of caviar turned out to be something of the same. For me, on a one to ten scale, champagne ranks as a one, while salty caviar might hit a four.

- As I moved into my forties, I found my body could no longer tolerate some of the foods I had been eating just from habit. I began to be intolerant to certain foods and to have reactions. I tried to ignore this, but the reactions became worse. At first these experiences happened almost immediately after eating certain foods. As I became even more sensitive, I found that just thinking about having a certain food would cause the same reaction I would have from eating it! These reactions varied at different times and with different foods: having a flushed face, a runny nose, stomach cramps or feelings of great tiredness. I underwent a test that confirmed that many of the foods I had experienced and had *thought* were the problems actually *were* the problem. I had just not been listening to my body (which had been speaking to me very loudly). The test told me to cut out things like wine, salt, sugar, tea, coffee, and chocolate - all of which I had loved, but which were doing me no good (confirming the reactions I had already had to these items). When I followed this advice, my health (energy) improved immediately.

- Some symptoms can also be a positive sign of the body's effort to detoxify – which it does when we have a cold – and may not necessarily be a sign that the food we have just eaten was wrong for us. Sometimes switching to a cleansing diet may trigger these kinds of symptoms for the first few days.

- I went out to dinner at a friend's house. They had asked me beforehand if I had any preferences, and I said no, as I had assumed she had roughly similar tastes to mine. When I got there, I found she had prepared one of my least liked dishes and I ended up being able to eat just enough to satisfy politeness. I made a decision to be clearer about preferences in future.

Shaun
- I thought the highest foods for me were tasty ones with rich sauces, but on testing for texture, feeling and taste, I find these foods aren't really my best ones (except occasionally), and that more natural ones, such as grains, pulses,

vegetables and fruits actually do taste and feel better, and retain a firm texture even when cooked.

- It wasn't enough to check out taste and textures, but also how it feels in the stomach - or later - does it feel heavy, or does there feel like there will be some other discomfort or negative body reaction?

- Foods, which are 'number ones' for us, change with the seasons, or with our geographical location.

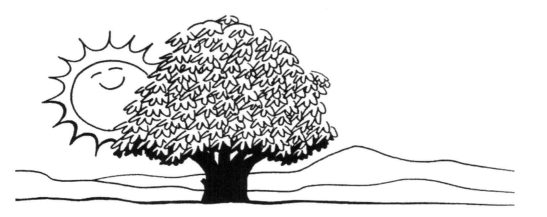

CHAPTER 4

Love What We Eat

The third principle is loving what we eat: chewing our food, tasting it, enjoying the different qualities of different foods and taking our time over it. This meant finding and savouring the sweet and the sour, the salty and the bland, the aromatic and the pungent, the astringent, the bitter and the fragrant, along with the different colours and textures different foods have.

Some associate love with 'duty.' This principle is about enjoyment, passion and an active feeling of gratitude for what we are eating. The time food spends in the mouth is the time we enjoy it most (and it is during this time that the mouth is stimulated to produce saliva that will aid digestion).

This principle is about loving everything we put into our bodies as the divine energy food is and realising that whatever we ingest we are transmuting from something outside into energy for our body's well being.

By blessing our food, we raise its vibration. By eating it with gratitude, we dwell on its benefits for us. Making food a celebration not only improves our enjoyment of it, it also improves our digestion.

When we stop loving what we are eating, it is time to stop eating, which brings us to Principle 4...

Our Experiences and Comments

Shaun

I found I was often hurrying the meal or eating without any awareness of what was going in. It's just food, I thought, and it's time to put some in the body. An opportunity to enjoy a meal was missed. The most enjoyed and memorable meals are the ones I eat slowly and with awareness of each mouthful. I remember to this day a flight to South Africa 15 years ago when I took an hour to eat the airline meal, chewing each morsel thoroughly. It was a brilliant meal, though the content wasn't an obvious choice or anything special. When I take time to enjoy a meal, my body responds pleasurably.

Brian

- I increasingly realize that what I think about food affects how I feel about it and how my body reacts to it. My body has reduced energy when I eat something I know may be beyond its 'use by' nutritious life. Conversely, if I am having something that is very fresh (whether it cost a lot or not), I feel more vibrant.

- The more conscious I grow, the more it has also become clear to me that who I am with when I am eating and what is being shared in words and feelings have profound impacts on my enjoyment of what I am eating and my feelings of its benefits.

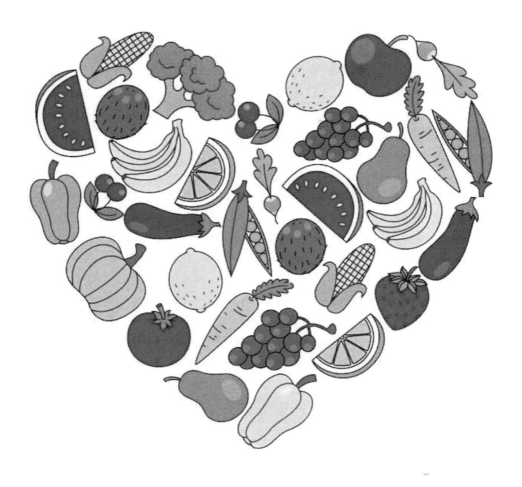

CHAPTER 5

Stop When We Have Had Enough

The fourth principle is stopping when we have had enough. We found we often didn't listen to that voice in our body that told us, "That's enough." Even if we did hear this message, we were more likely to say, "Wait a minute! I just bought this whole cheesecake. It cost me money and I am going to get it all in!" The little voice inside was telling us, after only one or two mouthfuls, "That was nice and tasted good, but that's enough."

We were trained from childhood to finish what was on our plates, sometimes because we were told it had been paid for with hard-earned money, and sometimes that not eating it would somehow be disrespectful to the starving masses. How our eating things we did not want would help others, we had no idea, but this was the programming many of us had. It can be fine to clean our plate, but if we are not hungry, eating it will not do anyone any good. Unless you package what's on your plate and send it off to the starving, finishing what you are not hungry for doesn't help anyone ...least of all yourself.

There are many social reasons why we eat beyond the point of loving our food and of having enough. Two major ones are good manners and consideration for the starving. This is particularly true for people who were raised during a depression, a war, other times of food scarcity or of food rationing. It becomes a "think of the starving people" issue in which not eating all the food in front of you necessarily implies waste and ingratitude.

Another reason we may not stop once we have had enough is when stopping brings on feelings of panic and an anxiety that we will be hungry again soon. If these feelings come up, it is important to be reassured there will be food available for the next time we may want to eat. Also, for those having these feelings, it is important to eat when reaching a moderate state of hunger, rather than waiting until feeling ravenous.

When we learned to stop when we had had enough, we found we began allowing ourselves to have more of the things we loved, just because we knew we could stop when we had had a sufficiency. For example, if we love chocolate, but have had a normal pattern of eating a whole box of it, we might have denied it to ourselves for that very reason. Once we train ourselves to eating a piece, while being conscious of its taste, texture and flavour, and really sucking on it and chewing it (rather than swallowing piece after piece while watching television or reading a book), we may well find we have had enough after one or two pieces.

Learning to stop when we have had enough with one of the foods that we love can be the beginning of mastery over that particular food, and an enjoyable mastery, too, for now we know we can have another piece tomorrow or whenever else we want to. It becomes one of our highest rated foods, or a number ten, which we now allow ourselves to eat.

Our Experiences and Comments on Stopping

James
I feel it's a waste when I do not finish what's on my plate. I became aware of how much I go for comfort eating and a full feeling.

Shaun and Harriet
- We both had experiences at restaurants where we found we had had enough after just eating the starter, even though more had been ordered. Now we feel liberated to have just a starter at times when eating out.

Shaun
- I get the inner signal "That's enough," but it's often when I am halfway through the first course and I think, "I can't possibly stop now. There are two courses to go!" So, I override the signal, suffer from feeling overfull and the body has to work extra hard to process the meal. I realise that I don't need the volume of food I eat and that somewhere I have been programmed into eating as a way of life, a way of social contact and as a time-filler.

Brian
- If I overeat, I prefer to do it consciously!

CHAPTER 6

The Essence of Nutrition

The essence of nutrition is energy. Food is only one of the mediums through which our bodies can acquire energy. From our experiences and discussions, we classified the main sources of energy as follows (from finest to grossest):

A. Foods of the Earth:

1. Direct products of the earth, including fruits, vegetables, seeds, nuts, pulses, grasses, seaweeds, herbs and spices. We found these foods are more easily transformed into energy (especially in their raw state, but also when only slightly cooked) than fish, animal or processed artificial, and sometimes part-synthetic, man-made foods.

2. Fish, which we found to be less dense than meat from animals.

3. Animal foods and products made from animals (such as eggs, milk and butter).

4. "Man-made," or "man-adjusted," foods that have been devitalised through processing: nutrient stripping, additives, spicing (to mask unpalatable flavours), irradiation, overcooking, and chemical treatments (to preserve) and what is laughingly called 'refining.' 'Refined' food is usually another word for "stripped of nutritional value." In observing our friends as well as characters from history, those who eat and ate the 'refined' foods ("meant for aristocrats"), usually are and were the least healthy. Our intuition also placed foods that had been interfered with through biotechnology, or genetic modification in this category.

B. Other than "Foods of the Earth" Categories

1. **Divine Spirit**, *Prana*, or pure nutrition, without which we wouldn't exist. This may also be awakened through the nourishment we receive in the form of love and joyful practices, like coming together in intimacy, meditation, prayer, the energy which comes from being in love (when food may almost seem superfluous) or that feeling which comes from just being in the presence of loved and loving ones.

2. **Air**, which affects us not only through breathing with our lungs, but also through our skin.

3. **Water**, through both drinking and bathing. As with air, we feed with water not only through our mouths, but also through our skins. The degree of nourishment will vary with the quality of water. The experience of fresh and clean mineral water felt better to us than water that had been treated, or maybe even recycled.

4. **Fire** - the energy from sunshine, fire and other light, the former of which is the source of energy for direct products of the earth. Fire was invariably recognised as one of the greatest and finest transformers by traditional peoples of the world. Many Westerners and Easterners today have forgotten the value and magic of the living flame.

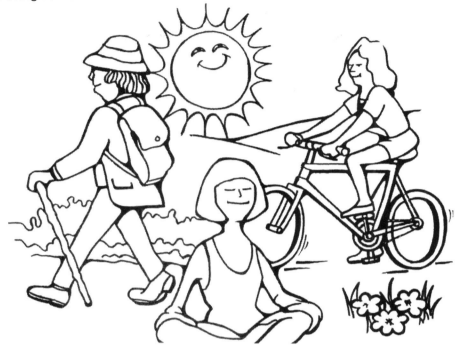

There are many other forms of nourishment not mentioned in the broad categories covered above. Some of these include the other nourishment received through other than taste senses - smelling (the fragrance alone of flowers and of delicious foods), hearing (uplifting music), touching (hugging, love-making, massage and what the skin receives through massage oils), sight (colours, beautiful scenery and the sight of loved ones), feeling (being open to and receiving harmonious vibrations) as well as nourishment the body receives through any supplements we may be taking (orally, inhaled, through the skin or even as a suppository), none of which, however, are the subject of this book.

It is worth keeping in mind that staying conscious is also being aware that nourishment isn't just about food and a few vitamins in our mouths; it includes all the senses. If we are deprived of any of the other forms of nourishment, we may try incorrectly to fill those needs through eating. Often what we thought was a call for food was a call for emotional nourishment - love, intimacy, connection, touch, acknowledgement - and filling that call with food was only a temporary solution that didn't answer the call correctly. This raises the larger issue of emotional and spiritual nourishment, upon which we touch later.

The key revelation that we found from our exploration is that eating consciously cannot be separated from living consciously. Indeed, our experience has been that practising the former may well begin a process toward the latter.

Further Experiences and Comments

Harriet
- I have tried and recommend a fast on water in which vegetables have been cooked.

- Our attitude to food and eating is a huge part of the process. I have heard the psychologist Victor Frankl made the decision he was not starving but fasting while he was in a concentration camp and this decision helped him actually feel there were benefits to that situation.

Brian
- Feeling good about what I eat and gratitude for it makes a huge difference to my digestive process and how I feel after eating.

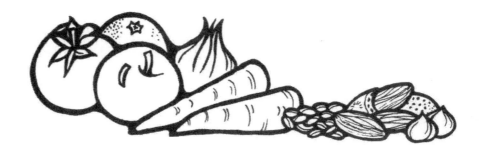

CHAPTER 7

Self-Exploration - YOUR Programme

The eight stages of self-exploration exercises outlined below can inspire you to develop your own personal conscious eating (and enjoyment of nutrition for life!) programme. They can be done over eight weeks, with one stage per week, or whatever shorter or longer period suits you individually. You will find some can be practised simultaneously with others, especially the earlier ones when doing the later ones. While they are meant to be sequential, feel free to combine however many of them you are comfortable doing together.

It is important when doing these stages, to have awareness on the body and its feelings, rather than on our traditional way of letting our thinking run our lives. The four principles need to have your body's awareness and energy brought to them for them to be followed successfully.

However, remember that the purpose of this book is to inspire conscious eating and its consequent wellbeing, rather than to make anyone feel they have to follow any rigorous set of instructions. You are completely free to use all, some or none of the steps below, to mix some of the stages with whatever works for you or to develop an entire programme of your own.

Stage 1 – What and When Do I Eat ...and Why?

Bringing awareness to your eating habits and patterns is the beginning of conscious eating. Many people eat unconsciously (are not, or are hardly aware of, eating), especially when snacking.

For a week or two (or more) keep a food diary, noting what you eat, the time, where you are, how hungry you were when you started and finished and a 'comments' column on thoughts or feelings you had just before or while eating which may have triggered the eating.

The foods you eat can be graded from "one" to "ten," with the "one's" being the foods you least like and the "ten's" those you like most. Make your list of the foods you feel are number "tens" for you. Try to be as specific as possible within the various food categories, such as fruits, appetisers, soups, salads, main courses (which vegetables and which meats, or what other sources of protein), desserts, snacks, juices and/or other drinks, noting also if you prefer the food raw or cooked. You may find it helpful to keep a separate list by category and to include seasonings, herbs and spices on your list(s).

You may also wish to note in your food diary how each item rates on this personal "one" to "ten" score card (or, better, how it rated as a "one" to "ten" when you ate it). Check to see what percentages of scores were "nines" or "tens," at the end of each week you keep this diary. This is a good indication of how willing you are to give yourself permission to live the 'good life.'

We found that we often rated our 'binge-type' foods as "tens," but put what our body was telling us was wholesome down to bottom ratings.

Your food diary will help you become aware of and able to respond to the following questions:

"Did I eat because I was hungry?" If not, note the reason. Example reasons can include:
- "I had some space left in my stomach."
- "I was in the kitchen."
- "I had guests (who were - or were not - hungry)."
- "It would have been impolite to refuse."
- "I was raised always to eat at this time."
- "It was left over and would have just gone to waste otherwise."
- "I was frustrated/angry/tired/depressed/in need of comforting."
- "I deserved a reward."
- "I couldn't sleep."
- "I was celebrating."
- "I eat when I am not hungry ...and to hell with the conscious eating programme!"

(Note: if you do this last one, it probably reflects an authority conflict. So, ask yourself, "Who do I think is controlling me?")

"What are my eating slots?"
- "Do I eat once, twice, three, four or more times a day, or do I eat constantly ...and do I really need to?"
- "Do I eat nothing all day and then pig out in the evening?"
- "Do I starve myself for several days and then overeat?"
- "When do I have my main meal of the day, and how do I feel after it?"
- "When, and how much, do I snack on?"
- "Do I have different eating patterns on weekends than I do on weekdays?"
- "Do I eat differently (more or less, or at different times) when I eat out than when I am at home?"
- "Do I take time to eat (and, if not always, do I enjoy eating more when I do)?"
- "Do I allow space/time for digestion?"
- "Do I eat differently when I am in company than when I am alone (and what's the difference)?"

"What foods do I eat most, which ones least ...and why?"

You may also be able to start answering the question of "Where do I experience hunger?" Watch your body! Are you really hungry or is it just a craving? We found we did not experience hunger in the stomach. There is an actual hunger, a psychological hunger and a hunger created by chemicals (as occurs when experiencing withdrawal symptoms).

In keeping notes about your eating habits and reasons for eating, we cannot recommend strongly enough that you do so as dispassionately as possible, without letting them have you form any judgement about yourself. Such a diary is solely for your private use (unless you choose to share it). The objective is just to achieve awareness, not judgement. Our own experience has been that bringing awareness just on its own to the above issues has gradually assisted in shifting us towards a closer adherence to the first principle: eat when you are hungry.

If you continue to keep your food diary beyond the first couple of weeks, it is likely you will find the foods you eat changing and your level of enjoyment in eating increasing.

Our Experiences and Comments on Self-Exploration

Shaun
- There is family karma around all aspects of life, including food - we are programmed with beliefs from our parents.

Brian
- I am aware that I may skip breakfast or only have fruit when I am at home. However, if I am staying at a hotel where breakfast is included in the room charge, I will tend to have a full cooked one. Although I do reduce my food intake during the rest of such days, my energy in the morning usually suffers, as much of it is drawn off in the digestion process.

Stage 2 – What Do I Really Love Eating

In this stage you discover what your real number "tens" are by testing the foods from your Stage 1 lists, along with all other foods you eat. You will probably find your list of "tens" changes dramatically, either immediately or just over a more gradual period of time. You may, for example, have thought sausages were a "ten," but it now turned out they are a number "one" or "two." It was only your head saying they were a "ten."

Eat your foods with as much bodily awareness as possible (keeping your mind and its judgements out of the way). This testing includes an appreciation of colour, smell, texture, freshness and/or the degree the foods have been cooked or not ...with care and aware chewing before swallowing.

> - Are your "tens" really as scrumptious and nourishing as you thought they were?
> - Do you feel a difference in the amount of energy different foods give?
> - Do you find that some of what you thought were "tens" are actually "supposed to eat" ones that came from childhood training in "good" and "bad" foods, and that these ones really rate well below a "ten?"
> - Do you find that other foods that you thought were "tens" for as much as you could get of them, are actually "tens" only for a little and, if you try to eat more, they actually turn into "fives" or less? (For example, "I used to find three bars of chocolate good, but now I find that one or two squares from one is plenty.")

Do I deny myself some foods (especially if they are "tens") ...and why? Are there particular beliefs I have about these foods or about my worthiness to have them? Do food prices influence my choice of foods?

Do my patterns of preparation influence what I eat and how high it scores? For example, do I tend to:
- prepare and home-cook my meals?
- use prepared meals bought at a supermarket?
- order take-away food?
- eat out? or,
- usually have microwaved food?

Does where my food come from, or the ways it is prepared, reflect the amount of time I am willing to devote to the enjoyment of eating?

After answering the above questions, adjust your list of "tens" accordingly, removing those you just previously thought were "tens" and noting which of the remaining ones you are quite happy with only a modest amount of.

Society's general conditioning about scarcity means that most of us, given the chance, gorge or overindulge on the things we value, often on rare occasions with long periods of abstinence in-between.

Others never let themselves have what they really like when they are alone.

We each have our own personal quirks concerning the foods we eat …and those we don't.

From this conscious testing, finding out that we really do like something, but in moderation, we can now give ourselves permission to enjoy it in smaller quantities …and more frequently!

One's list of "tens" may change all the time. A "ten" today may not be a "ten" tomorrow but may well become a "ten" again in three weeks. **Intuitive eating is a moveable feast!** But, in addition to "tens" you may well enjoy having several "nines," "eights" and "sevens" in your diet as well, especially when this means having them instead of your "ones," "twos" and "threes" which you may used to have felt obliged to eat.

The awareness that comes from this conscious testing moves us closer towards aligning with the second principle: Eat what you (**really**) love eating.

Our Experiences and Comments on What I Love Eating

Harriet
- I found I have two lists: a lazy/comfort B list (chips and omelettes) and a healthy A list. Realising this, I now want to eat consciously when having fantastic food, as I am now aware when I am full and can stop. However, I am not ready to completely let go of the B list …yet.

- I go from the A to the B list depending on my mood. Sometimes I find I'm 90% healthy (on the A list) and 10% not (on the B list) and at other times I'm the exact opposite. Negative feelings lead to the B list.

- I'm now conscious that when I eat biscuits/cookies, I am going for the double fix of salt and sugar together

James
- I now give myself permission to eat anything. I have also become more aware that I often do not really like what I have habitually been eating and don't enjoy what I am eating (but I haven't made the shift from this yet).

Brian
- I have a friend who is in his mid-nineties and who says food is his last great pleasure. He has been through rationing consequences of both World Wars. What he eats can sometimes seem appalling from today's medical guidance, yet he is in fairly robust health and still *really* enjoys shopping, preparing food and eating. I've often been tempted to recommend he improve his diet, but then wonder who is teaching who here…

Stage 3 – Eat Consciously All the Time

This stage is about extending Conscious Eating to all of your meals and snacks, including those you have away from home and on the run. Following it well will help you to learn to eat consciously, which includes chewing your food well.

A good way to keep your awareness and body consciousness on how well you are doing here is to resume or continue your food diary (when you eat, what you eat, and a "one" to "ten" score on each item, plus a 'why' you are eating and your thoughts and feelings before and/or when eating). If you have moved from relatively unconscious to more conscious eating, a comparison with the notes and diaries you kept from the first and second stages may be very revealing. You may even want to include and use a "zero" to "ten" barometer of how conscious you have been when eating. A very thorough approach could include a use of four barometers:
- hunger level when you started eating,
- 0-10 on your preferences for the foods,
- your degree of enjoyment, and
- you could even rate your level of consciousness (level of clarity about intuitive connection with body awareness).

The especially interesting comparisons will be between your times and frequency of eating now compared to your records from the first stage and the percentage of "nines" and "tens" you eat now compared with your diary kept during the second stage (and in how what you thought were "nines" and "tens" have changed. Having more "nines" and "tens" in your regular diet doesn't necessarily mean overindulgence in unhealthy and "forbidden" things. When you eat consciously (listening to your body), you are giving it the balanced and nutritious diet it really wants ...and may well also be giving the nutrients it needs to combat a condition of ill health. (Babies are naturally conscious eaters. An American test in which they were presented with a tray of many different foods showed they naturally chose for themselves foods which gave them a balanced and nutritious diet.)

It will be interesting to see what you call a "ten" now compared to what you thought was a "ten" in Stage 2.

Besides noting the when, what and its score in your diary, the most valuable aspect of this stage is to record honestly what triggered the desire to eat. *If it is not real hunger and you are honest about what it was, this awareness alone will be a **giant** step forward on your journey toward a Conscious Eating for life programme.* An awareness of our non-hunger reasons for eating is the beginning of our being able to come to terms with and resolve any unfinished issues for which we may have been eating as a way of compensation.

If you want to do this stage conscientiously, and yet find yourself in circumstances in which you are not eating as consciously (with awareness) as you would like to, WAIT TO EAT until you can remember yourself. In most circumstances it is possible to eat consciously whenever you can remember (be aware of) yourself. You are the only one who can give yourself a pass mark on this or any other stage of Conscious Eating.

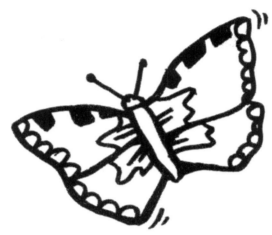

Stage 4 – Eat Adventurously!

Prepare Your Meals Consciously and Discover New Restaurants More Consciously.

Be adventurous with new foods! For the average Western diet, there are actually usually hundreds, and often thousands, of foods that have never been tried. Now's your chance!
Try
- new flavours, foreign foods (Mexican, Chinese, Indian, Middle Eastern, Japanese, Thai, Indonesian, Malaysian, French, Italian, German, Spanish, South American, African and many others),
- raw foods instead of cooked,
- different presentations and/or different food course eating sequences,
- preparation in new ways (such as with a wok, bamboo steamers, barbecue, fondue pot or tandoori oven), and for other changes
- try eating with chopsticks, or with your fingers.

When there is no time, having a take-away meal, or putting a pre-packaged meal into the microwave may do sometimes (some of our group had reservations about microwaved food), but for a Conscious Eater a very large part of the enjoyment of eating can also come from consciously preparing the food. The choice and freshness of ingredients, your creativity reflecting your individual preference in ingredients, along with the love you put into the preparation, can often be experienced as being as nourishing, if not more so, than actually eating the meal.

You may discover you reach a place where you can love yourself enough to cook well for yourself, as well as that place where you can really consciously receive and enjoy the preparations others prepare for you.

The first exercise here is to prepare your meals consciously for one week (even if it is only for one of your meals per day ...and however simple that meal might be). You may also wish to keep a note of the recipes that are number "tens" for you for future reference.

It can also help to prepare meals with friends. Compare lists of "tens." Exchange opportunities for cooking for each other.

Make Conscious Eating a joint adventure!

Exercise/meditation to bring about mindfulness in connection with a food:

Be mindless and come into the body ('lose your mind and come to your senses'). Put a little bit of fruit or nuts on a table in front of you, such as tangerine segments, grapes, walnuts, or pecans. For a moment, forget you have a mind that thinks you are a particular someone with a collection of past experiences. Just focus on the reality of the body's experience now. Become aware of the temperature, of something you see, the taste in your mouth, the smell in the air, the sounds you hear. Stay aware of these sensory experiences. The mind pretends to take ownership of these, but they are all just separate sensations belonging to no one at all. Now pick up the fruit or nut you have in front of you. Take a moment to become aware of what it feels like (its hardness, softness moistness or dryness), and see the colours and shapes it has. Smell it. Put a small piece into your mouth and savour its taste for a moment before chewing slowly and swallowing.

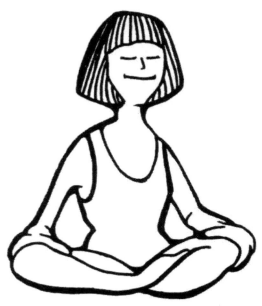

These sensory experiences (without any ego or personality owning them) are reality. You are not reading or thinking about eating. You are not watching someone else eat. You are not worried about yesterday or preoccupied with tomorrow. You are here and now, and the full appreciation of the food is happening within your greater awareness right now. You are eating consciously. Traditional Japanese haiku poems and Zen koans are experienced and written from a state like this, one where the author has stepped out of being the thinking mind and come back to conscious awareness of the body's sensations.

Our Experiences and Comments on Adventurous Eating

Harriet
- I am usually too busy to take time to cook, so instead I choose carefully when shopping and preparing ready-made meals.

Brian
- Living in Japan helped me appreciate the importance of food colours and presentation. This has become an important part of Conscious Eating and enjoyment for me.

- When I prepare food consciously, I am amazed at how beautiful and sensory it is – for example, the colours and branches on cauliflower and broccoli, the concentric rings in an onion, the segments of a citrus fruit, the colours of a fresh cut papaya and the amazing smells of fresh foods, herbs, and spices.

- Lama Surya Das's book *Awaken the Buddha Within* includes an eating meditation in which he advises the reader to sit, take a breath, feel thankful, and then put a few raisins - or something else similar which you have available - in your hand. Feel their texture, examine their colours and shapes, smell them, and then have a little taste (much as a wine connoisseur will consciously appreciate and sample a rare vintage).

- When I am in touch with my body, I can hear its call for the nourishment it most wants. I can come out of my mind with its identifications with past emotions, psychological states, compulsions, and obsessions. As I continue with this practice, I am also becoming more aware of the finer sense of intuition that helps guide me in food selection in the moment.

- As I moved more and more into intuitive eating and the intuitive preparation of foods, although I still used recipes to guide me about some food preparation, I would also get intuition to add other ingredients (especially spices). To double-check my intuition, I would smell or taste the new ingredient, before adding it, and have found this to be infallible, and a marvellous way of enhancing the dishes I make. I also follow intuition on the amount of any spice I add ...but often taste to test, as is a habit with any seasoned cook. Now I find I am fairly clear on what and how much of anything to add without the smell or taste test, but still enjoy the sensory experience. (WARNING! *I love spicy food.* While what I add to a recipe intuitively may be perfect for me, it may not always suit others who might be sharing the same meal. I have found I can also be intuitive about what will be best, or at least work well, for all when preparing a meal for others as well.)

- I have had many comments back on how great some food I have made is after I have consciously LOVED making it. *Putting love into the food we make makes a difference for everyone who shares it.*

Gill
- Last night we had an old friend over for supper and he had a <u>very</u> conscious meal. Crudité with humous to start; followed by baked salmon with prawns and tomato and flavoured with dill, lots of garlic and black pepper; accompanied by steamed vegetables, onto which he enjoyed pouring extra virgin olive oil. Afterwards the men had mince pies (a seasonal touch), whilst I had cheese. I felt very conscious of the way I had cooked the meal, more intuitively than usual, taking plenty of time to prepare everything with consideration and love. Shaun and our guest were very complimentary, and I felt good.

Stage 5 – Choose and Select Your Foods Consciously

As every successful restaurateur knows finding, selecting and buying your foods is critical. There is little point in preparing a meal with second- or third-rate ingredients ...and even less point in eating it with any real enjoyment or conscious nourishment.

This Fifth Stage invites you to extend your Conscious Eating back to even before the preparation stage, so that you consciously choose for yourself what you will be preparing and nourishing yourself with.

The exercise here is to visit markets, farms with foods for sale, the growing number of natural food stores and organic produce available, markets, greengrocers, butchers, grocery stores, supermarkets, or other food outlets *you feel best about*, and to select your food and other ingredients as consciously (listening to your body and intuition) as you can.

If you have time constraints and find it difficult to buy and prepare from the best ingredients available, select top quality prepared meals that you really feel are a treat for you.

As you make your choices, stay in touch with your inner barometer(s). Note the colour, smell, and feel of the food. Feel for the energy the food may have for you. Do not select food because you have to eat, because you've always been told such and such combinations are 'good' for you, or because you feel it are important to 'stuff' yourself. Be sensitive to what will nourish you and your well being.

Some find it is best to eat locally grown, rather than (out of season or exotic) imported, food. This may have to do with freshness or the body's alignment with similar energies or vibrations the food has from being grown where the body is also established. Others have a preference for food or herbs grown by themselves where this is possible - they had put their own energy into these foods and what could be fresher?

An additional part of this adventure is to explore regional and ethnic foods and to experiment with potential new and old number "tens" with the changes in foods that comes with the changes in seasons.

Our Experiences and Comments on Choosing Foods

Brian
- I find I prefer daily shopping, rather than every few days, weekly or with even longer gaps, to tune into my body's call now (but I still take advantage of special offers I feel good about). Freshness is important to me, as well as listening to the body to choose the food on the same day it will be consumed. I find myself using my freezer less than I used to.

Stage 6 – Celebrate Eating!

The most important aspect of eating is to enjoy our food. The more we enjoy it, the greater the energy we will have from it ...and the healthier we will be. This principle is one of gratitude and is reflected in the almost universal tradition of offering a blessing for a meal before it commences. It is also evident from many once-a-year celebrations around the world that honour the beneficence of nature and the harvest. North American's autumnal Thanksgiving is only one of innumerable examples of this. The practice of blessing, or saying grace, is a way of creating an enhanced feeling of gratitude for the gift received, raising its vibrations and thus increasing the nutrition of the food.

When we consciously choose and buy food and prepare it with love, we are naturally more aware of its energy.

This stage is about remembering yourself (being conscious and aware in your body) each time you eat and about feeling gratitude. You may not necessarily say a grace before a meal (which is a "thank you" for receiving God's grace or mercy), but there will be a sense of thankfulness about what you eat.

The important thing about restaurants or parties is ambience, where everybody is having a good time; laughing, talking, sharing and enjoying the food ...all of which is good for real nourishment and digestion. If you are eating alone, treat yourself as your best guest. Celebrating food is celebrating and honouring you.

If you do this stage conscientiously (and consciously!), it is unlikely you will be eating anything that is less than an "eight" on your scorecard. Succeeding in this stage means you have achieved the third principle of Conscious Eating: Love What You Eat.

Our Experiences and Comments on Celebrating Eating

Harriet
- There is an importance in honouring the food we eat. When we are on the run, or watching a movie or TV, eating chips hand to mouth may be mechanical, rather than conscious. Even though I was alone at times, I found it was important to eat sitting at a table. Otherwise, as with chips, hand to mouth eating was more often mechanical, rather than conscious.

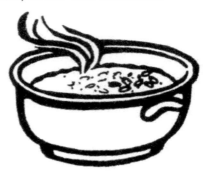

Stage 7 – Advanced Testing of Foods

In this stage you will learn that when you are conscious (aware in the body), you will find that when you are in a shop or at home, you can pick up and hold any food, imagine you have eaten it and feel what it would feel like ("How would I feel having this food inside me? How truly nourishing is this food for me now?").

You will have a sense of whether it is right for now (the next meal or snack), or better left for another time. Sometimes what is a "ten" in our scorecard is right for breakfast, but not for lunch or dinner. This sense, and bodily awareness, will help you select the nourishment that is right for you ...and reject those foods that do not serve you just now. You will have a sense as to what is right now ...or best left for another time

If you listen to your body, it will tell you what type of food it wants (savoury, sweet, bitter, or salty, as well as which texture ...but then test this for yourself!).

As you become more conscious and aware of your body's messages, you will find you don't need to pick up and hold a food to find out if it is right for you just now. Without even having it to hand, you can visualise eating whatever food you can imagine, and check with your body as to how nourishing it would be -- and your body will give you an immediate response. This is also the best way of making a choice from a menu. (Homeopathic practitioners rely on this method for selecting remedies.)

This advanced testing through visualisation has another major benefit. When we are sick or unwell, we can use the same method of reconnecting with our body to check which food would be the most healing for us at this time. This is also the time when we might be most sensitive. Each body is individual, and what is required for healing a body is individual. As regards nutrition, the Number One expert is you.

(However, if ever you are in doubt about these ways in connection with any health issue, please consult your doctor, practitioner, or nutritionist.)

Stage 8 – Stop When You Have Had Enough
(...and what to do When You Don't)

The fourth principle of Conscious Eating is to stop when you have had enough. Listen to the body and it will tell you when this is. What we have found is that the body tells us when we have had enough, but we often ignore it and continue eating. This principle is about respecting the body's messages.

Conscious eating cannot be separated from conscious living. If we eat more than what we want just from hunger, it is important to tell the truth about why we are eating more than the body really wants. (This is equally true when we deny ourselves food when legitimately hungry - what is the real reason behind why we are not eating?)

If you find you don't stop when you have had enough, be aware that you alone can make the choice.

Ask yourself, "If I have cravings, what do I lack?" Cravings may signal a call from the body for remedial nourishment, but if it is a situation of eating more than when you have had enough, there are usually aspects of compensation or compulsion involved.

Some example questions you could ask yourself about this:
- "Am I unsatisfied with some aspects of my life (and which ones are they)?"
- "Is food a substitute for love or sex for me?"
- "What am I avoiding?"
- "What am I holding on to?"
- "Why do I need a wall between myself and the world?"
- "What am I afraid of (what is my next step)?

It is important to address the issues that come up for you in this stage. Being conscious (having an awareness) about what triggers eating for you and about what moves you on to eat more than what satisfies natural hunger will usually lead you to those unresolved issues in your life which have been driving you to eat, or to deny eating, as a form of compensation. An issue with eating is invariably a metaphor for an issue one has with life in general. Being conscious allows you to watch for the patterns.

There are underlying causes to not stopping when we have had enough that are worth exploring. The main question to ask your self is "What causes me to eat when I have had enough?" Such thoughts could be:
- "It's wrong not to clean the plate."
- "What about the starving in Africa?"
- "I overeat to please my mother."
- "I don't know when I will get another meal, so I might as well fill up now."
- "I feel safer when I am stuffed."
- "I can't sleep on an empty stomach."
- "I deserve some pleasure in my life, and food is one of my main ones."

This is a good step for self-enquiry. If you stop when your body has had enough, but you still want more, see what comes up for you.

The exercise here is just to be increasingly aware of those subconscious or unconscious behaviours, which may have been running your life, and to start addressing them in new and nourishing (but other than eating, or avoidance of eating) ways.

If you are aware you eat in a compulsive, or even addictive, way, we recommend doing this programme with a support group (and calling on medical or other support as required). It may take some time but go for healing the underlying issues and for more conscious and balanced eating. Be self-accepting, rather than self-judgemental. *There is no need to be perfect!* Just aim for more balance and conscious awareness around eating. Also, always remember that conscious eating is about tending more and more to normalcy and natural nourishment, and *never* about having a restrictive diet mentality.

Eating consciously leads to living consciously. As you place attention on eating consciously, you will begin to discover that it cannot be separated from living consciously since, as you bring a conscious awareness to your body, you automatically bring a conscious awareness to your life. You will find you will also want to clean up your relationships and clean up your life, so that you have in it the things that truly nourish you.

We wish you well on this adventure!

Our Experiences and Comments on Advanced Testing

Katya

- Before, whenever I didn't feel comfortable in my body, I used to check what I was eating and make resolutions like, "Right! As of tomorrow, I'll start to eat healthily - just raw fruit and vegetables" ...but this never worked. Now I say, "Okay, in which ways am I not fully expressing myself?" This way I am using any discomfort in my body to find the real roots underlying the feeling. My body becomes my buddy! This approach allows me to see how I can really support my body and myself by consciously choosing food that is more nourishing and which reflects my true love of myself. This means I now find myself naturally eating more healthily, and yet still enjoying enough of all the foods I want to eat.

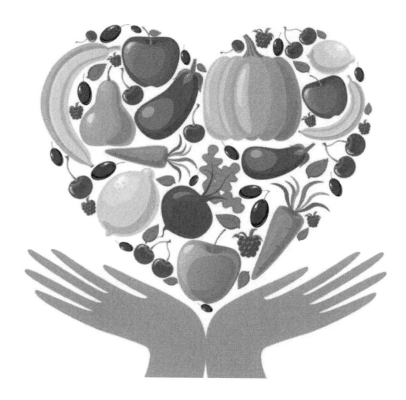

CHAPTER 8

Questions and Answers

Q. I have very little control over what I eat. Can this programme help me?

A. Yes. The traditional approach is control and domination (e.g., diet and denial). This actually creates a counter-reaction of indulgence. Conscious Eating suggests an entirely different approach - one of love and awareness in our relationship with nourishment. Thus, love and what we really enjoy eating leads the way.

Q. What if I don't really want to eat?

A. Don't eat. Trust your body. Take care that you are listening to your body, rather than to your mind or emotions. Not being nourished as a result of conditions like anorexia or bulimia is not about *not* really wanting to eat, but more about self-concepts based on misjudgements from the past. Be clear that when you don't want to eat, that is really a message from the body or, perhaps, a conscious decision to fast for reasons that will enhance health and wellbeing. (If in any doubt that not eating will be a health concern for you, check first with your doctor, practitioner, or nutritionist.)

Q. Will I get different energies from different foods?

A. Yes. Each food carries its own frequencies, and the body calls for different frequencies at different times (as you will know, for example, from how your tastes differ in summer from what they are in winter). There is no set formula, however, which applies to everyone.

Q. What about eating late at night?

A. Conscious Eating is not telling you what or what not to eat, or when or when not to eat it. It is about asking you to follow the four principles. Make your own choices.

Q. What if I have little time for eating and, as a result, have poor digestion?

A. You have just answered your own question. If you were to eat more consciously (following the suggestions of this programme) your digestion would almost certainly improve. You would be well advised also to explore why you give yourself so little time for eating.

Q. What do I do about addictions like alcohol, coffee, tea or chocolate?

A. These are covered by the principles: Eat when you are hungry (not when you are anxious or compensating); Eat what you love; Love what you eat (eating or drinking with love is not doing the same with compulsion/addiction); and stop when you've had enough (when what is true hunger is satisfied). If you are not able to hold to these principles around an addiction that is health threatening, we recommend you seek specialist assistance from some of the wonderful organisations that exist to provide help and support in these areas.

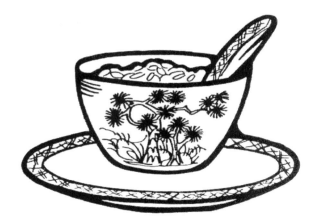

Q. Is vegetarianism a better route than eating meat?

A. We make no judgement on what is better for you. The conclusions we found were individual to each of us. Similarly, your preferences will be found through Conscious Eating and practising the principles. You may well find, while eating consciously, that nature's foods come very high on your list of preferred foods and that these foods feel better. Test for yourself. What are the most nourishing and enjoyable foods for you?

Q. How do I know I am getting this right?

A. Conscious Eating is an exploration, not a "getting it right." Trying to "get it right" puts great stress on you. Our interest is that you test the principles and discover the most enjoyable and nutritious way of eating for you. Your body's call and response is your best teacher.

Q. What if I crave certain things?

A. A craving can be a natural hunger and the body's voice speaking to you. Make the distinction between a craving and a compulsion or an addiction. A compulsion or an addiction is not conscious. A pregnant woman craves certain things, but this is a call of the body, rather than an addiction. We may answer a craving with something which does not satisfy the body's real call (for example, if the craving is for sweetness, eating chocolate cake or sugar may well just create more craving, whereas you may find that if you have a natural sweet, like fruit, that may satisfy the craving. The test is, "Has what I have eaten satisfied the call?"

Q. What about eating processed and fast foods?

A. Test these foods against the principles and make your own choice.

Q. Can I lose or gain weight following the Conscious Eating programme?

A. Yes ...as you truly eat consciously you will find your body weight adjusts to what is naturally correct for you.

Q. How long do I do this for?

A. This is not a diet. This is a new approach to eating for life based on love - the love you have for yourself and for your body. You do it for as long as you choose.

Q. What about taking medicines or vitamins while eating consciously?

A. This programme is about a conscious approach to eating. Any medicines or supplements you take on top of this are again a question of listening to your body, as well as a matter for discussion with your doctor, practitioner, or nutritionist.

Q. Should I continue the Conscious Eating programme if I am not feeling well?

A. Yes. When the body is feeling unwell, it is even more sensitive to what it wants in nourishment, textures, and tastes. Illness can often have an emotional base. As we become more aware of our bodies, we become more conscious of the tensions and stresses we have ...and we can start to release those with love.

Q. What if I am eating at social occasions and have no choice which foods I eat.

A. Eat consciously anyway. It's what you do in the majority of your eating which counts, rather than on exceptional occasions. A Conscious Eating programme is a guide meant to assist you, not to create more problems for you. On such social occasions, choose what you love to eat best from what is available and enjoy it. Revert to full conscious eating at your next meal, or as soon as you can.

There may still be times when you consciously choose to have a blowout or a special occasion ...and you will find that you can even eat consciously while having a blowout.

Q. What if I stop before I have had enough?

A. Some people prefer to be a little bit hungry to keep themselves alert. This is your choice. The fourth principle is to stop when you have had enough. If you are in doubt as to whether or not you have had enough, wait a while (like 5 minutes) to recheck with the body to see if it is satisfied or not.

CHAPTER 9

Summary Results for Us

When we REALLY experienced eating what we thought were our number "nines" and "tens", we frequently found that many of them dropped down to "threes" or "fours." Our memories told us we loved them, but our experience told us we didn't, and a number of foods we had previously thought as low on our list became "nines" and "tens."

By eating consciously, we began valuing present experience more than what memory is telling us.

Most of us found we had valued certain foods and drinks for years just because others valued them, or because they were expensive. When we sampled them in the light of our present experience, we often found we they were just 'so-so' or that we didn't like them at all.

Similarly, when our experience of something was that it tasted disgusting, felt disgusting and - for us - had no life energy in it, we chose either to stop eating it or to reduce the quantities of it we ate -- and not as a deprivation, but because we really preferred it that way. (These included times when we would previously have eaten some or more of something purely out of 'politeness.') We found we could leave *whole* food groups out without experiencing any adverse effects.

Conscious eating leads us naturally to transform our eating, rather than find we have to control it or to deny ourselves those foods and drinks we love.

The test is to experience with our full consciousness (in the experience of the now, rather than just in the mind and/or the emotions) what it really is we DO like to eat and drink ...and if we really do like something, it becomes something we can allow ourselves to have *consciously*. This way there isn't any effort, denial, control, eating when we are not hungry or "*having*" to finish things when we eat anymore. It is allowing us to be conscious and loving ourselves enough, and our bodies, to use these simple principles.

Most importantly, the awareness practiced in Conscious Eating can be an invaluable means to reconnect with our own spontaneous inner intuition, inspiration and guidance, so we no longer have to feel dependent on outside books, teachers and other influences. No one outside us can have a better understanding of what is truly better for us than our own inner guide, or Higher Mind. With this guide as the observer, we are also no longer slaves to our mind, our ego with its psychological patterns or to our emotions. And through this observer's awareness, we can well find that Conscious Eating extends into other parts of our lives ... until we discover we are truly *Living Consciously*.

Our Experiences and Comments on Our Results

Harriet
- I did a similar programme before which worked very well. In it I first had to accept myself and I also combined conscious eating with an exercise programme at a gym. I lost nearly thirty pounds in about a year.

- I found myself going through four stages with this conscious eating programme: first binge eating; next eating crap, but increasingly aware of it; thirdly gradually dropping some of the things I was eating, but which my body wasn't calling for; and, finally, moving into relatively eating consciously virtually all of the time.

Shaun
- I find the programme does away with all the beliefs around controlling our eating; "I mustn't eat this; This is fattening; This isn't good for me." These self-terrorising thoughts give way to an awakening to awareness of what my body and mind's natural choice is. Certain foods and drinks drop away without effort and I'm left with a greater freedom to eat or not eat and to enjoy my choice of food whatever it is.

Gill
- I was excited at starting the Conscious eating programme and doing it with others also provided the support I needed to get going. There have been many times before when I have been more conscious of what I consume than what I normally have been ...periods of being vegetarian, two 10-day brown rice fasts, and when only eating raw food. So, I started this programme with confidence. However, during the days which followed, I found myself unconsciously eating snatched meals; being given chocolate, buns, and other foods I would not normally buy (but ones I love to indulge in); and being invited to parties and boozy lunches (fun, but distracting!). I was well into the second week before I re-focussed and started spending more time in both the preparation and eating of food.
There are three of us at home. Shaun and I are both eating consciously, while eleven-year-old Danny, who eats what he wants, is probably more conscious than both of us. He eats exactly what he likes and is often seen cooking his own meal. His diet includes all the usual yummy fast foods enjoyed by his age group yet, unusually, also includes a wide variety of salads and green vegetables.

- I recently found myself alone for four days, and I didn't go near a supermarket. I went to our local greengrocer's store and really considered what I wanted to buy and eat. I bought a variety of fruit and vegetables and a loaf of wholemeal bread. I had no desire at all to have meat or fish, which I do enjoy. All I wanted for the weekend was toast for breakfast with tea, fruit (particularly bananas) for lunch and a large plate of steamed vegetables for supper, covered with the best Italian extra virgin olive oil and a little tamari sauce, so its salt could bring out the flavour of the vegetables. During this time, I found I had plenty of energy and enthusiasm for a good clear out in my office AND to lay the kitchen and bathroom flooring in the flat! Since then, I have wanted to follow the same eating pattern. I'm choosing vegiburgers (without buns) and salad or a sandwich for lunch when working away from home, and oatcakes, unsalted nuts and crunchy bars for snacks.

Katya
- The most important insights I got from my involvement with the Conscious Eating project are the following:
- How I relate to food, and to eating, depends on how I feel about myself.
- My body size and weight and how I feel about my body is independent of what and how much I eat.
- My eating is closely linked to my level of self-expression. The more freely I express myself, the less I find I need to store in my body.
- This awareness helped me change my attitude to eating.

- Before, whenever I didn't feel comfortable in my body, I used to check what I was eating and make resolutions like, "Right! As of tomorrow, I'll start to eat healthily - just raw fruit and vegetables" ...but this never worked. Now I say, "Okay, in which ways am I not fully expressing myself?" This way I am using any discomfort in my body to find the real roots underlying the feeling. My body becomes my buddy! This approach allows me to see how I can really support my body and myself by consciously choosing food that is more nourishing and which reflects my true love of myself. This means I now find myself naturally eating more healthily, and yet still enjoying enough of all the foods I want to eat.

- Using the principles of Conscious Eating helps me put my awareness on which foods I enjoy most while eating, in terms of flavours and texture, and on how energised I feel after having certain foods. I put the best ones in the upper ranges of my list of "tens," which I like to have to hand when next shopping.

Brian
- It is a joy to have the awareness Conscious Eating brings – to shop consciously, prepare foods with awareness and love, and eat just the amount that feels enjoyable and satisfying. I find I now eat less than I used to, but it is usually better quality and I enjoy it much more. My diet varies more, too, as I am spontaneous in what I choose. This makes food an adventure, as I rarely know ahead what will be next on the menu.
- What is also wonderful is the way this awareness and spontaneity increasingly spills over into other aspects of my life, making more and more of my daily life more and more of an adventure.

[**NOTE**: If you try the programme and keep notes on your findings and want to share them with us, please post such comments in reviews. We truly welcome all such feedback and will consider including those in a possible revision, either with your real names or anonymously, as you prefer.]

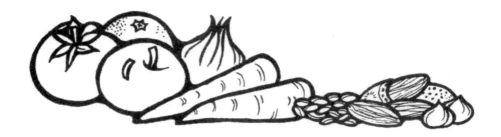

REALLY Loved Foods   **Ranking out of 10**   **date entered**

Food Diary Week Number

Date Time   Food   Ranking out of 10   Eating Reason

_____

_____

_____

_____

_____

_____

_____

_____

_____

_____

_____

_____

_____

_____

_____

_____

_____

_____

_____

_____

_____

_____

_____

_____

_____

_____

_____

_____

Food Diary Week Number _____

Date Time   Food   **Ranking out of 10   Eating Reason**

Other books by Shaun de Warren

You are the Key – A Guide to Self-Discovery

"Shaun describes his work as 'holding the vision of Oneness and assisting people to manage their lives in all its aspects from this viewpoint and with joy and ease.' A wonderful book of spiritual exposition and one which I would ardently recommend." - Brian Graham, Science of Thought Review

The Mirror of Life – Your Adventure in Self-Discovery

"It's very interesting to watch 'out there' to find out about ourselves . . . I radiate thoughts that are bouncing back in the mirror of life so that I can see them . . . the fascinating thing is, if we make our adjustments here in what we see 'over there', we find that 'over there' changes."

Money Mastery *(with Rosalind de Boland Roberts)*

"This book is an invitation to create a new relationship with money. We are shown that the barrier to abundance is found in our personal beliefs with which we have been programmed since birth. The key to unravelling our limiting beliefs lies in aligning ourselves with universal laws that are not only lucid and simple, but accessible to everyone. A practical guide with real stories that illustrate wealth creating principles."

Your Wellspring of Plenty – Let Go the Cupful and Have the Ocean

"How much more prosperity, happiness, joy, wealth, abundance and love can I take? Being our prosperous selves is exciting, fun and easy. This practical psycho-spiritual book with sections on 'It's all yours for the asking', 'Loving yourself', and 'Tapping into your inexhaustible well of plenty' shows you how."

From Pitsville to Joyville
The Harris Visits the Garden of Everything
(Illustrated by Gill Coupland/de Warren)

Compilations (with illustrations and design by Gill Coupland/de Warren)

The Prosperity Handbook – Gems to Enrich Your Life and Pocket
The Relationships Handbook – Jewels to Bring Love and Happiness
The Health Handbook – Pearls to Inspire Healing

Other books by Brian Mayne

England's Festivals – A Year of Seasons, Customs and Traditions

"This was a completely unexpected discovery. It's a delight to dip into, month by month. I'm learning all sorts of things about English customs and traditions. Thoroughly recommended." – John Wormald

Who Am I? An Exploration of Our Essential Nature

An illustrated discovery document exploring what our essential nature is . . . and is not. Is the waking state our true reality? Does who we are begin and end?

CONSCIOUS EATING
An Invitation to Intuitive Nourishment

A group of us, dissatisfied with diets and confused by what all the "experts" say on what we should and should not eat, came together to explore a different way ...a way directed from within and a way which trusts that the body knows what it wants and needs if we truly listen to it.

Conscious eating is about becoming aware of the call of the body, which speaks to us intuitively, rather than through the mind or emotions. The body, we discovered, calls for love and for nutrition created from love. The mind and emotions are subject to habit, compulsion, and addiction, which are not love.

Our group expanded into more than one and these were made up of different individuals with a variety of occupations: management consultant, publisher, author, counsellor, university professor, graphics designer, performer, beauty therapist, financial controller, mothers, and homemakers (of both sexes) among others.

Thus, we embarked on our journey, basing it on four simple principles we had discovered.

We invite you to participate in this experiment and we recommend you try the programme included here. Each stage of it is intended to inspire, support, and take you to deeper and deeper levels of exploring what conscious eating means for you.

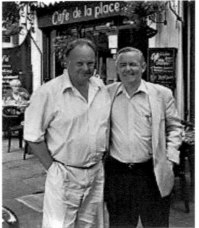

Shaun and Brian, Battersea, 1999

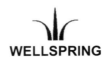

WELLSPRING

Printed in Great Britain
by Amazon

85951809R00029